C000097389

THE BOY IN THE MIRROR

The Boy in
the Mirror

Tom Preston

Valley Press

First published in 2015 by Valley Press
Woodend, The Crescent, Scarborough, YO11 2PW
www.valleypressuk.com

First edition, first printing (August 2015)

ISBN 978-1-908853-53-0
Cat. no. VP0070

Copyright © Tom Preston 2015

The right of Tom Preston to be identified as the
author of this work has been asserted in accordance with
the Copyright, Designs and Patents Act 1988.

All rights reserved. No part of this publication may be
reproduced, stored in or introduced into a retrieval system,
or transmitted in any form, by any means (electronic,
mechanical, photocopying, recording or otherwise) without
prior written permission from the rights holders.

A CIP record for this book is available from the British Library.

Printed and bound in the EU by Pulsio, Paris.

www.valleypressuk.com/authors/tompreston

For all those who were there,
and those who have been since.

Breathe in and hold your breath.

You're lying on your back, arms raised above your head, your whole body perfectly still, air held uncomfortably in your lungs.
Breathe normally.
You feel the dye rush through your veins and your mouth tastes like metal. Here comes the hot flush. He said it might feel like you've passed water.
Breathe in and hold your breath.
Your eyes are drawn to a little red line under the glass. A sign reads, 'Do not stare directly at the laser.' You look away.
Breathe normally.
The whirring slows and comes to a stop.
Breathe normally.
Breathe normally.

Back in the waiting room, the scene is all dressing gowns and slippers. Zippy anoraks and woolly cardigans. Sad eyes.

They give you a queue-jump. A little red ticket. 'What service!' your dad says, half-joking. You manage a weak smile; the faster they see you, the worse your chances are.

Results will take up to three weeks.
They call you at home three hours later.
Can you come in today? We need to talk about your CT scan. Any time is fine. Any time you want.

The consultant's office is all scribbles and charts. Academia. His eyes are warm, peering over his glasses. He talks about numbers and percentages. Your mother and father don't move at all as he speaks. Not even slightly.

Breathe in and hold your breath.

The nurse stands behind him, arms folded, her face a picture of comfort and reassurance. Her eyes twinkle with sadness; she knows how bad it is.

Your consultant says, 'The next step is called a PET scan. It's a kind of nuclear medicine that produces a 3D image of the inside of your body. It can detect and pinpoint hypermetabolic activity. I've booked you in for first thing tomorrow. It should tell us exactly what's going on.'

Hold your breath.

It's a cold, blue morning and you're standing in a car park on your own next to a huge grey mobile building. A careful man in a white uniform gestures for you to climb the stairs. Inside, they sit you down and the mood is faux-joviality. Trivial words.

This scene is all computers and clinical waste disposal bins.

'We need to put this into your arm.'

The dye flows through the cannula into your veins but this time it doesn't feel weird. The man tells you the nuclear dye means you are now temporarily radioactive. He leaves the room.

Over the intercom his voice crackles. 'You need to wait here for a few minutes before your scan. They'll call you in. Just shout for us if you need any help. When the scan is finished you'll need to wait a few minutes for the radiation to diminish. After that, you can go. For today, avoid pregnant women and animals. Just as a precaution.'

Eight-thirty the next evening. You're standing at the bar in a cheap pub buying a round of drinks for you and your friends. You interrupt yourself as you order with a brief coughing fit. It sounds terrible. The barmaid looks at you oddly.

'You ought to get that checked out!'

You smile, 'I know.'

It's at this point you touch your throat and notice the hard little lump on the side of your neck. Something rushes through you, not quite panic, something else – something closer to the feeling of falling.

On the Ear, Nose and Throat ward the mood is boredom and tension. The scene is all flimsy hospital gowns, anxious checking of watches and ruffling of newspapers. The waiting room is just you and three older men, maybe in their fifties or sixties. In the corner a TV silently cycles through the early morning news.

The surgeon comes in to explain your operation. It's relatively simple and should take little more than an hour. First they're going to make an incision along your neck just under your chin. Then they're going to carefully cut out the malignant lymph node and the sample will be sent for analysis.

There is a slight risk at this point in the operation that one of the delicate nerves in your neck may be severed. This could result in an asymmetrical smile or difficulty eating after surgery. Such damage would be permanent.

At the end of the procedure the surgeon is going to drill into your pelvic bone, take a sample of marrow, and see if the disease is present there. Both stages of the operation will be performed under general anaesthetic.

You're taken to a holding room and asked to lie on a raised bed.

This scene is all children's cartoons and comforting pastel paintings.

The anaesthetist puts a needle into the back of your left hand. He asks you to count down from ten. Your eyes blur and the world swims around you.

You awake in a room, it could be the same but you can't be sure.

The scene is unclear.

Your mind soars and you laugh. Though you don't quite understand why, something is very funny.

You float into a lift and feel infinitely comfortable as you descend, and you sleep.

The next time you wake you feel happy but fuzzy. Lifted but heavy. You're in a bed on the ward and you can hear the soothing sound of your parents' voices from behind the curtain. They're talking to the consultant about something. About you. You drift in and out of their hushed exchange.

PET scan showed advanced spread of disease.

12cm tumour in the chest cavity pushing against the trachea, causing cough.

Tumours also present in neck, lungs, kidneys, spleen, bowel and bones.

Assumed diagnosis is high-grade diffuse large B-cell lymphoma, stage four.

Optimistic prognosis would be somewhere around 40%.

'Cancer is a word, not a sentence.'

You're back in the consultant's office the day after surgery. You're here to discuss your options. The bone marrow sample confirmed the initial diagnosis, he says. There's a poster on the wall featuring a smiling young man with very short hair. 'Jonathan had acute myeloid leukaemia – after two years of chemotherapy, he is now in remission. Cancer is a word, not a sentence.'

Your consultant tells you there's a new medical trial being run at the City Hospital. It's an intensive regime of chemotherapy that packs a year's worth of treatment into four months. You'd need to live in the hospital as an in-patient during this time. He's spoken to the haematology ward there already. You can move in tomorrow.

He tells you this is your best chance.

The City Hospital is around seventy miles north of home.

You are faced with a choice: either stay home with your family and friends and receive outpatient treatment at the local hospital, or move away from them all and live in isolation on the ward at the City Hospital until hopefully you get better.

There's no time to think about this decision.

Your consultant's words echo in your head: 'This is your best chance.'

You call your friends and tell them the news. You arrange to meet them in the pub for one last drink.

The pub is all wipe-clean upholstery and waterproof menus. At the bar you're served by the same barmaid who commented on your cough last week.

'How's that nasty cough?' she asks.

'Not great,' you reply, but you smile.

As you turn your head her eyes flick to the large white surgical patch on your neck. She looks away quickly and goes to get your change.

Back at the table the mood is all stubborn optimism and good humour.

Your friends seem brittle but brave all at once. One friend holds your hand under the table as they ask questions about chemotherapy.

You don't have many answers.

The next morning you visit a fertility clinic before you leave for the hospital. The chemotherapy will most likely make you infertile so the NHS is going to store a sample in a sperm bank so you can still have children in the future.

The scene in the waiting room is all anxious couples and vases of flowers and home-keeping magazines.

A nurse asks you some questions and takes some blood. She gives you a plastic pot and leads you to a room with a small sink, a clinical reclining bed with a tissue-paper cover sheet, and a black cabinet containing NHS-approved pornography. The pornography is laminated.

Back at home and you're packing a bag for hospital. Books. DVDs. Photographs of people you love. Pyjamas.

Your mum walks into your room and looks at you sadly.

'You'll probably get through loads of books!'

Downstairs you stand with your parents and sister in the kitchen. You realise how much you love them. Nobody knows what to say. Your dad draws you all together into a hug. The scene is all wet eyes and sniffing back tears.

'I'm so sorry,' he says, his voice cracking just a little, the three of you held tight in his gorilla grip.

'You'll be okay.'

'You'll be okay.'

The haematology in-patient ward is all bright lights, beeping machines, business-like nurses, and a complete absence of patients. Each room is private. The communal area is deserted. This is where you sit with your family while they sterilise your room.

A nurse brings everyone teas and coffees. After a few hours, your sister suggests a walk. You walk with her quietly round the hospital corridors. It smells of cleaning products and old furniture.

Eventually your room is ready. Everyone says their goodbyes and you're on your own. It's late, and you're tired.

The soft lighting and fresh sheets make the room seem like some bizarre hotel. You catch a glimpse of yourself in your bathroom mirror; you look pale and shaken.

A nurse comes in and puts a cannula into the back of your left hand then hooks you up to a fluid drip. He leaves and you go to undress but you can't take your shirt off because of the tube from your hand to the drip. You settle for pyjama bottoms and curl up into bed.

The ward is peaceful but for the gentle patter of shoes and the far-off beeping of a machine in a room somewhere else.

You sleep.

You're about to feel a sharp scratch.

The next morning you're woken by the same nurse who hooked you up to the drip the previous evening. It's dark in your room.

He's here to take some blood.

'You're about to feel a sharp scratch,' he says.

The nurse ties an elastic ribbon around your forearm and pushes a needle into a vein on the back of your wrist. It stings a little. Small test tubes with plastic tops are popped into the end of the syringe and one-by-one are filled with blood.

He uses a trolley equipped with different instruments to measure your temperature, blood pressure and oxygen absorption rate. He asks you if you urinated during the night. He asks you if you were able to empty your bowels. He records everything on a data sheet attached to a blue clipboard.

This is called observations, he tells you. Once you start chemo, they'll be doing them every six hours.

'What if I'm asleep?' you ask.

He smiles. 'Then we wake you up.'

Your new consultant comes into your room and introduces himself. By now it's late morning.

He's all scruffy hair, complicated-looking numerical tables and warm, thoughtful smiles. With him are two other people: the specialist lymphoma nurse and a haematology registrar. They explain how your treatment is going to work.

There will be four cycles. Each cycle lasts a month. The first and third cycles are the same regime of drugs; the second and fourth also mirror one another. The hope is that by the end of the fourth cycle the disease has responded.

Your consultant doesn't mention what happens if the disease does not respond.

Chemotherapy will be administered by specially trained nurses through something known as a Hickman line: a catheter surgically inserted into your chest and connected to the superior vena cava. This allows instant, safe, intravenous administration of the chemo and also quick access for blood-letting, infection control and pain management.

On eight occasions during treatment a doctor will inject chemotherapy directly into your spine.

These are called intrathecal injections, or lumbar punctures. The purpose of this is to protect the brain against the development of cancer. The intravenously administered chemotherapy cannot reach the brain or spinal cord due to the blood-brain barrier so these injections are a necessary part of your treatment.

Your doctor tells you that many people find these injections particularly unpleasant.

He tells you that there will be significant side-effects to the intravenous chemotherapy regimes and that these side-effects may be more severe because of the intensity of this medical trial.

The side-effects may include: nausea, vomiting, total hair loss, loss of bladder control, loss of bowel control, fatigue, loss of appetite, hot rashes, skin-shedding, mucusitis, infertility, severe internal pain, nose bleeds, and a substantially weakened immune system.

He tells you that you will need to be kept in hospital for the duration of these four cycles. Depending on how you respond, you may be allowed home for a day or so at a time to be with your family.

He tells you to get plenty of rest while you're feeling strong.

He tells you you're in the best place you can be.

Tomorrow you will be fitted with your Hickman line.

Tomorrow you will start your chemotherapy.

Your parents come to visit in the afternoon. Prior to starting chemo you've been given a course of steroids.

The predominant side-effect is hunger.

After months of tapering appetite and awkwardly uneaten meals, suddenly you cannot stop eating.

You feel alive to the possibility that drugs really can change your body; quietly this gives you some faint sense of hope.

NHS food comes in branded blue and white packaging. Tuna and cucumber sandwiches in a blue and white cardboard box. Carrot soup with two blue and white packets of salt. Roast dinner. Sponge pudding with custard. You eat it all with grateful, childish fervour.

The woman who brings your food is bright and kind. She's friendly and you feel at ease. She brings you a clear-plastic jug with a green top.

'This is your two litres of water. You're expected to drink this much every day.'

She smiles and places a small stack of 250ml plastic cups on your table.

'Just take it one cup at a time.'

Your parents come in and the woman leaves, smiling at them as she goes. They see you've eaten a whole meal and eye you suspiciously, smiling.

'It's the steroids,' you tell them.

They sit down, one on each chair; you return to your bed, dragging your drip with you, and sit cross-legged on the blue and white sheets.

A medical machine behind you beeps like a metronome.

'We've brought you some stuff,' your dad says.

'Just a few things to make it feel like home,' your mum adds.

She takes out a selection of pillows and blankets and busies herself placing them around your room.

Your dad has a large cardboard tube that contains some posters from home. Film posters. Music posters. The same ones that you had on your walls when you were a student, just a few weeks before.

'It'll be just like you're at uni again,' he says wryly.

Your parents have just met your new consultant; they've been briefed on the medical trial and the structure of the treatment.

They ask you how you're feeling and you're honest: aside from the cough and some strange pain in your stomach, you feel okay. They seem pleased.

They brought you some biscuits. You talk for a couple of hours. About family. About home.

This time when they leave it isn't so late at night and you're not so exhausted.

You don't want them to go.

You're reminded of that first day at university, which seems so long ago, their eyes filled with pride and hope as they left you. Back then, when they closed the door to leave they seemed at the same time to open up to you a world of exciting, scary, unknowable and endless possibilities.

Today, as they close the door, their eyes clouded with fear and sadness, you feel numb and alone.

You watch them from behind the blinds of your window as they walk to the car, your dad's arm wrapped tight around your mum, their heads clenched together.

You watch them until long after the car has gone and the sun has set and you're stood alone in the darkness, machines beeping softly in distant rooms down silent corridors until at last you have no choice but to tear your eyes away and climb into bed, familiar faces smiling down at you from walls above.

The registrar comes to your room early the next morning, just after 6am observations, and disconnects your drip.

He tells you that today you won't be eating. You're going to be given a sedative to relax you when your Hickman line is fitted. Sedatives affect your digestion.

'When will the operation be?' you ask hungrily. The steroids are still giving you an artificial appetite.

'Before 2pm,' he says. 'Try to get some sleep.'

The woman who brings your food comes to your door a couple of hours later. You see her image swim towards you through frosted glass and blurry morning eyes. She stops and reads something on the door, turns around, and leaves.

You summon the energy to climb down from your bed, feet curled on the cold floor, and open the door once she's gone. The registrar's note reads, in scrawled handwriting, 'NIL BY MOUTH.'

You return to your bed and pour yourself a plastic cup of water from yesterday's two-litre jug. The water tastes like metal.

Trees dance outside your window but the thick glass renders the wind mute.

These windows can't be opened.

Across the grass and beyond the car park an old couple huddle by a bus stop, shielding each other from the chill.

You look at the time, pull the sheets up to your chin, roll over, and try to sleep.

A man in green scrubs comes to your room. You aren't sure what time it is. He has uneven stubble and a large, kind face.

'Time to go mate,' he says. 'You ready?'

A second man, tall and awkward, comes into your room behind him with a wheelchair. You climb down from your bed and into the chair. It is only once the second man is pushing you out of your room do you realise that you don't actually need a wheelchair at all – you feel okay today. But you're tired and hungry and anxious and you're too embarrassed to say anything now so you let him push you through the ward and into the lift.

The first man asks how you're feeling. You tell him you're tired and he nods. His face is lined with compassion. You feel like he wants you to be okay.

Your journey through the hospital bursts with misery and noise. Children wail and cry. An elderly man shakes and moans, delirious. Visiting families huddle for comfort like animals starved of warmth.

You do not yet feel like you are a part of this.

In the theatre they help you from the wheelchair onto a bed. A nurse asks you to remove your dressing gown and pyjama top. She rolls them up and places them by your feet. She pulls the blanket up to your chest and hands you a small paper cup, just like the one for your pills on the ward. It contains one large off-yellow tablet. She hands you a plastic cup of water.

'It's a sedative,' she says. 'It won't put you to sleep, but it will help you to relax.' She speaks efficiently. She doesn't smile.

'The surgeon will be making two incisions: one in your neck near your jugular vein, and one near your heart. He'll then push a tube from the bottom incision under the skin to meet the one at the top. This is your Hickman line. It will let your doctors and nurses give you chemotherapy quickly and safely.'

She speaks as if from a script.

Your eyes are drawn to an old lady with very pale skin; she is wheeled out from the theatre and back to the waiting room. A curtain is drawn around her.

The nurse carries on. 'Most people don't experience too much pain, but you will find it quite uncomfortable, almost like the surgeon is pushing too hard – this feeling is normal.'

The nurse walks into the theatre and calls something to the surgeon. She returns. 'We're ready for you.'

The Hickman line procedure takes about fifteen minutes. The nurse was right: it's uncomfortable, but not particularly painful. It's unpleasant enough that you wish never to have to do it again.

Back on the ward, your chest and neck hurt. They feel bruised and the tube under your skin is tight.

Uncomfortable and unnatural.

You check the time on your phone and realise that soon they'll be bringing up your food. You smile to yourself at the value of simple pleasures and unconsciously caress the weird worm that now lies resident in your chest; a new part of you.

By the time the registrar comes to your room it's late and night time has bleached the hospital ward with the eerie glow of artificial light. He attaches a saline drip to your Hickman line via a blue box that regulates the flow of fluid electronically.

'This is just to prepare the line for the chemo. I'll be back soon.'

Several minutes later the registrar returns and is followed into the room by the same nurse who hooked you up to the fluid drip on your first night. The nurse is pushing a yellow trolley with 'CYTOTOXIC WASTE' printed in large black letters on the side.

The registrar is carrying a metal tray upon which sits a dark brown plastic pouch. He asks to see your Hickman line and you lift up your shirt. He peels back the surgical patch and the nurse peers over. They nod at one another; the nurse begins to prepare the dark brown pouch. As he does this, the registrar explains what's happening.

'This is your first dose of chemotherapy. The infusion will take around two hours. Once it's complete, someone will come to disconnect the drip. You won't notice any immediate side-effects, but you will probably want to sleep afterwards.'

The nurse attaches the plastic tube coming from your Hickman line to the brown pouch. He lifts the pouch up above his head and hooks it to the top of the drip stand.

You watch, transfixed, as the first droplet of chemotherapy bubbles from the bottom of the pouch and wobbles above the fluid in the drip line.

Neither the doctor nor the nurse say anything.

The scene is tense.

Your eyes stay fixed on the bubble of chemo.

It drops.

And there it is. Some drug. Some drug you will never fully understand; some drug that may well play a role in saving your life.

Nobody on the ward, in the hospital, or in any hospital in the world, can tell you if this is going to work.

Nobody is qualified to predict with any certainty whether you will respond to this drug or whether it will simply torture you while the cancer kills you anyway.

Once you reach this point, there is no more science; there is only chance.

It was the roll of the dice that led you to this moment and it is only the dice that can save you now.

You are alone.

All that you have left is hope.

Just try to hold still.

You're lying on your side, legs tucked up into your chest, a pillow between your knees and another under your head, drenched in sweat.

The procedure has been going on for several minutes. You aren't sure how long exactly. You've been shaking for a while now.

This is your first injection of chemotherapy into your spine.

Before it began, a registrar came in to double-check the label on the drug. He nodded, left the room, and a second doctor started to ready the needles. As he did so, the doctor explained that only some chemotherapy drugs can be safely administered in this way; accidentally injecting the wrong chemo into your spine can be fatal. It's a very nasty and painful way to die. For that reason, every injection is double-checked by a second doctor. Just in case. The drug you will be injected with today is called methotrexate. It's one of the few drugs that can be safely administered through the spine.

Methotrexate was originally developed to induce abortion in cases of unwanted pregnancy.

A nurse is here with you. Her hand is on your shoulder.

'Just try to hold still. It'll be over soon.'

You're in a small room on the ward with a bed and a sink. The doctor is injecting the first, larger needle into the space between two of the vertebrae in your lower back.

The first needle is used to extract fluid from your spine. This is to ensure that a pathway has been found to the central nervous system – if the fluid is clear and contains no blood, the pathway is pure.

The second injection is smaller and is administered through the pathway established by the first needle. It contains the methotrexate.

Your doctor has injected the first needle into your spine seven or eight times now. None of the previous attempts yielded any spinal fluid. Neither he nor the nurse are sure why.

Some of the injections cause you significant pain. The needle touches against a nerve in your spine and sends a harsh, sharp signal all the way down the right side of your body. With each fresh attempt, you anticipate another shock.

The sweat pours down the back of your neck and onto the wet pillow.

You grit your teeth.

After the procedure you're led back to your room in a wheelchair and helped gingerly from the chair onto your bed. The nurse hands you a small paper cup that contains two 15mg codeine tablets.

'Take these,' she says. 'Your back will ache today. Try to lie still and get some rest.'

The codeine takes about twenty minutes to take effect. You aren't accustomed to prescription analgesics so you drift pleasantly into an opioid-induced sleep.

You awake feeling fuzzy.

A nurse stands over you.

You smile and your eyes half close.

Time passes.

Your friend has come to visit. She arrives just as the nurse is starting another chemotherapy infusion.

'Oh!' she stops. 'I'm sorry.' She seems embarrassed, like she's walked in on something private.

The Hickman line hangs loosely from your exposed chest. The wire runs up through the electronic regulator and to the nurse's hand as she hooks the bag over the top of the drip stand.

You smile fondly at your friend. It's good to see her: a familiar face in a strange new world.

The nurse leaves and the two of you talk for an hour or so about friends from home, family, the news. Neither of you mention cancer.

After a while, the drip timer beeps to signal the end of the infusion. The nurse reappears and detaches the empty bag of chemo.

Your friend says she has to leave. You don't want her to go. Suddenly, the prospect of the long night ahead, alone, seems frightening.

Silence hangs thickly in the air and you want more than anything else to ask her to stay for another hour. To talk to you about anything other than cancer and hospitals.

You look at your friend. Her eyes are damp.

Machines beep and click and a light rain dots the window. The air outside looks cold and fresh but in here it's dense and warm. Artificial.

She says it again. 'I have to go.' This time her voice sounds strained.

You nod.

She hugs you tightly and makes her way to the door, waving sadly as she goes.

A few days into your first cycle of chemotherapy you begin to lose your appetite. The thought of food makes you feel nauseous.

Your throat feels sore, like you've got a bad cold.

Water tastes stranger each day.

You find yourself wanting to sleep most of the time.

You drift in and out of the surreal pantomime of daytime TV, punctuated by six-hourly observations, business-like conversations with doctors, and the ritual of chemotherapy infusions.

Every few hours you are given a menu of assorted pills to regulate your weakened immune system, replenish your damaged blood chemistry, and manage your pain.

You begin to suffer from severe and sharp aches in your gut. This is normal, your consultant tells you, and he doubles your codeine dosage to 60mg.

Afternoons roll by, as the winter gales pound your window and the rain lashes hard on the roof of the hospital building and you submerge yourself gratefully into the warm sleep that codeine so easily grants you.

More time passes. Each scene is a postcard of solitude and slumber.

You wake late at night, the ward silent but for the hum of machinery, and walk your drip stand to the toilet.

When you turn on the bathroom light your reflection stares numbly back at you, gormless and vacant. You blink. Your eyes are yellow, as is your skin. You've lost weight: your pyjamas hang off your arms like the wilting leaves of a dying plant.

You stare at yourself in the mirror for several surreal minutes. The thing before you is not you. But it is.

Your skin itches and flakes when you scratch it from your arms. You wipe the dead skin from your bed sheet and it collects in a shameful patch on the floor but you're too leaden to care. You turn over and sleep.

The next morning your consultant comes in wearing a grim face. You prime yourself for bad news.

'Everything is normal,' he says.

Breathe.

This is the tension you experience every single day.

'Today we're going to start you on the high-dose methotrexate infusion. It's the most challenging part of the regime. We hook you up for thirty-six hours, then disconnect you and begin what we call "rescue" – that's where we flush it all out of your system with fluid. You'll need to urinate a lot during this time, so the nurse will provide you with a bottle.'

You nod. 'Why is it so challenging?' you ask.

'High-dose methotrexate can be very damaging. It hits your immune system hard and has several difficult side-effects. We'll deal with those as they come up. You need to be monitored every hour of the thirty-six hour infusion. We do this through obs. If your temperature spikes or your blood pressure drops too low, we start the rescue early. This infusion historically presents significant risk.'

You feel the colour draining from your face.

'Don't worry, you're in good hands. You'll be fine.'

The thirty-six hours pass mostly without incident. You lie awake for almost the entire time.

Every time you begin to drift off to sleep, a nurse or a doctor comes in and records your temperature, blood pressure and oxygen absorption rate on the observation chart.

This time the clipboard is red, not blue.

By the time the infusion is finished you're deliriously tired. Your eyes ache. Your body is heavy. You can't tell what is fatigue and what is chemo. Finally, the methotrexate is disconnected and the nurse begins your fluid rescue.

You sleep, but awake every few minutes to urinate. You

use the cardboard bottles the nurse provides you with, carefully doing so under your bed sheets to preserve your fragile dignity. You line the urine-filled cardboard bottles up along the floor by the bedside cupboard like obscene collector's items. Nurses come in wordlessly to take the bottles away every hour or so.

The second night seems to go on forever.

At some point you stop needing to urinate.

The grey light of morning leaks through the clouds and the chatter of a new day slowly grows in the background of the ward.

The scene is purposeful. Routine.

You sit up in your bed and feel quietly, sadly alone.

The pain begins in your mouth.

Then it spreads to your throat.

Then your insides begin to cramp and twinge and it feels like your gut is burning.

It's hours before the doctor is able to see you.

'Methotrexate can cause a condition called mucositis,' your consultant tells you, while you squirm in your bed.

'The chemo dries up the mucous membrane in your body and inhibits your ability to replenish it. Your mouth and throat dry up, as does your digestive system.'

You twist.

'This is what is causing the pain in your mouth, throat, and stomach right now.'

You turn.

'There isn't anything we can give you to stop it, but good oral hygiene can prevent infection and we can prescribe pain killers to make you feel more comfortable.'

You gurn. Your throat splinters.

You dab blood from the cracks in your lips; the broken blisters on the inside of your cheeks.

Even drinking water is painful. It slides down your throat like crushed glass. You hold every swallow for as long as possible, then close your eyes and grit your teeth.

In your head you imagine sandpaper. Serrated knives. Barbed wire.

For several days now, codeine has been your blanket. You slept under its gentle glow. Now, it doesn't even touch the pain.

The doctor prescribes oramorph – the oral morphine solution. It's sugary and pleasant. You administer it yourself via oral syringes. It helps the pain a little, but not a lot.

You try to sleep.

You haven't eaten in two days.

Nurses come and go.

Fluid drips and antivirals and potassium. Oramorph. Codeine.

People come to visit but you're tired and in pain. Their faces swim before you. Some visitors are turned away.

Blue-and-white labeled food is brought in on plastic trays and quietly removed an hour later, untouched.

The scene is all bloodied tissues and antibacterial mouthwash.

The scene twitches and shakes at the edges as the pain spikes and subsides.

You experience a growing need for opioids.

With the nurse out of the room, you take twice the dose of oramorph that you've been prescribed.

The scene fades into darkness.

The next morning the pain nurse arrives, asks you some questions, and leaves.

You writhe in your bed.

Soon after, she's back with a silver trolley housing an enormous syringe. The syringe is cased in blue plastic.

The nurse takes a key from her belt and turns it in the lock on the blue casing. The monitor beeps; high-pitched, almost shrill.

Written in black letters on the side of the syringe are the words 'DIAMORPHINE PUMP.'

Your eyes flicker.

You've read about diamorphine in the pain management pamphlet a nurse gave you. It's the chemical name for heroin.

'We'll slowly up the dosage every hour until your pain subsides,' the nurse says. The light from the lamps over your bed reflect in her eyes. She seems kind.

The pump is hooked up to your Hickman line. You watch in awe as the diamorphine slowly snakes up the tube and into your body.

The first hour passes and you're underwhelmed by the effect.

Your mouth and throat sting and burn.

Your gut cramps and twists.

Blood trickles from your nose and leaks from the sores in your mouth.

A hot, red rash burns on your arms and legs.

The pain nurse returns again and again, each time increasing the dosage. Eventually it reaches maximum: 5ml per hour.

You wonder if this happens to everyone.

You wonder if you will ever feel okay again.

The heroin flows through you pleasantly.

Eventually the pain begins to change – it stays, constant, but it's less important.

Dreams hang above you, misty and half-formed. Scenes from your childhood. Parks and swings. Board games on the carpet of your grandparents' house. Your little sister's face. There's laughter and bright colours, faded into grey.

Someone is here to visit. You don't know who. Images dance above you; indifferent memories.

Someone takes your hand and holds it tightly.

A voice resonates in the distance.

Then fades away.

Are you awake?

'Mum? Is he awake?'

Your sister's voice grows clearer and louder as your eyes slowly open.

The room is blurry.

She stands over you.

'Are you awake?'

Her eyes come into focus. They're wide and worried.

You croak a response. 'Hi.'

Your mum and sister have come to visit. You can't be sure what time it is. The room is light. The ward seems busy.

This scene feels familiar, almost homely.

You don't know how long you've been asleep. You glance over to the diamorphine pump. The display reads '1.5ml p/h.' The pain nurse must have reduced the flow while you were sleeping. You feel grateful for the lucidity.

'So how are you?' your mum asks, her face aching with concern.

'Okay…' you mumble.

You look around your room. The cardboard bottles of urine have all been cleared away. As have the bloodied tissues and discarded oral syringes.

A fluid drip has been attached to the second lumen on your Hickman line, so both diamorphine and saline are now flowing into your bloodstream.

Your mum places two packets of cookies on your bed-side table.

'For when you're feeling better,' she smiles.

You realise you haven't eaten in at least three days. Maybe four.

Scratching your head absent-mindedly, you notice how weak and loose your hair is. You scratch harder, pull out a small clump and hold it in your hand. You stare at it for a long time.

There's dead skin all over your bed sheets and dried blood on the inside of your mouth and nose. Your throat still throbs with pain and your insides still ache. The pain is becoming background noise.

Your sister seems nervous. You try to calm her down with talk of school, of friends, of TV.

Around you, machines beep and click.

Your mum seems calm. Both her children in one place, together.

This scene feels safe.

When they go, you don't mind. Something has begun to change. Some kind of acceptance.

You wave as they shut the door, sharing smiles. It feels important that they see you smile.

It's been a week since you ate any food. A dietitian comes to see you. He's very tall and thin. He tells you that because you haven't been eating, it's important for you to take on nutrition in other ways to keep strong and healthy. The fluid drip can provide some of the essentials, but energy has to come from food.

'Because of your sore throat, I'm going to recommend you drink these high-calorie nutritional milkshakes. They're banana flavoured.'

The dietitian asks you to climb down from your bed and walk over to the scales in your room. He has to help you down. You wince and grimace as you walk. Your legs ache from days spent immobile, and your gut burns with pain.

You stand, with help, on the scales. You've lost 12 pounds in the last week.

'This is a dangerous pace of weight loss,' he says. 'It's vital that you drink three of these milkshakes a day. And drink water whenever you can.'

He leaves and shortly afterwards a nurse brings you one of the milkshakes. They taste awful. Like salt. Like stale milk. You can't be sure if they're really this bad or if it's just the effect of the chemo on your taste buds.

The milkshake soothes your mouth but burns your throat. You think of broken porcelain. It takes a very long time to drink. Afterwards, you're exhausted. You top up the diamorphine with a dose of oramorph.

Sleep comes to you quickly.

Cold sun leaks through the window and you absent-mindedly pull clumps of hair from your head as you watch a grim-looking group of patients wait for the hospital bus.

The hair slips away from your scalp with ease, like slow-cooked meat from a bone. It's oddly satisfying. Sometimes you stop, just for a moment, and inspect the clumps before dropping them into a bin near your bed. Your pillow is littered with hair shed during the night. Like a dog's blanket.

You used to have a morning routine. Shampoo. Conditioner. Hair cream. Shaving foam. Aftershave. Products that made you feel clean and fresh; that helped you to shape your identity each day.

Now you sit in bed with huge flakes of skin peeling from your arms and neck, dried blood coating your lips and mouth, and clumps of your thin, fragile hair falling pitifully from your head.

Your morning routine involves chemotherapy and antiseptic mouthwash.

The boy staring back at you from the mirror this morning has pale, yellow skin and thin, greying hair.

He is not you.

He cannot be you.

He is you only in a desperate, vulnerable future – broken and old.

You take action against the indignity of your slow hair loss, the embarrassing thinning, weakening and shedding. You run an electric razor over your head. Again and again. Over and over until what remains of those fragile hairs is left scattered on the bathroom floor.

You look dismally at your own reflection.

A feeble caricature of yourself.

Bald and weak.

A cancer campaign poster.

An object of pity.

It's mid-afternoon and you're sat half-up in bed, intently peeling a long piece of skin from your arm.

It started as a little bubble up by your shoulder and with great care you've slowly peeled down to nearly your elbow without the peel breaking.

Eventually it tapers to a smooth break and the skin is left hanging, twirling bizarrely in your hand.

You finally exhale.

A doctor bustles into your room.

'Your temperature has been running a little high over the last couple of observations so we're going to send you for a chest X-Ray to make sure you don't have an infection in your lungs. With the chemo weakening your immune system, you're more susceptible to infections, and less capable of fighting them off. Bacterial chest infections might pose risks of more serious problems like pneumonia.'

The same men who came to collect you for your Hickman line implant help you into a wheelchair and push you to the X-Ray department. This time on the journey you drift into a dreamy fog.

Scenes are becoming repetitive.
You follow the lines on the floor.
Everything is background noise.
Lights above you flicker and hum.

They park your wheelchair next to an old lady. A voice overhead talks in monotone. *Dr Hayes to X-Ray please.*

The old lady is bald. Maybe she's not that old, just aged. Your eyes meet and she smiles widely.

'Snap!' she says, pointing to her head. 'I got one of those cuts!' Still smiling, she looks you up and down. 'Only I suppose you choose to have yours like that?'

'No...' you hold her gaze. 'Chemo. Lymphoma.'

Her face changes a little and she looks at you carefully. 'Bowel cancer,' she says eventually. 'It's my second bout.'

A soft silence hangs between you. This is the first fellow cancer patient you have met. The old lady holds up a plastic pouch. It's packed with pairs of knickers. She laughs: 'Just in case I mess myself! I've been there before!'

And you both laugh. Not nervously, or out of social need. Genuine, sincere laughter. At the absurdity. The baldness, the wheelchairs, the emergency underwear; the indignity of it all. The moment doesn't last more than a few seconds, but the two of you connect. Your misery and sadness and anxiety is momentarily washed away and you feel, with nauseating delight, like a human being again.

As soon as the laughter dies down, a nurse comes and takes the lady away. As she's being pushed towards the X-Ray room, she calls out and asks your name.

You tell her.

She tells you hers.

You both smile.

'Good luck,' she says. And she's gone.

Just sit tight.

At the end of your first cycle of chemo your consultant grants you a day at home. It's been a month since you began treatment. A month in which you've not left the hospital.

Your dad picks you up in his car.

This scene is all overnight bags and reassuring smiles.

He helps you from the wheelchair into the front seat. You're so tired you struggle to keep your eyes open.

Eventually the car rolls into your home town. Familiar signposts and buildings flash by. Your head aches and throbs.

The nurses packed up an enormous NHS-branded plastic bag full of your prescription drugs: antibiotics, antivirals and anti-sickness; morphine, codeine and paracetamol to manage the pain; powder for your high-calorie milkshakes; folic acid to counteract the side-effects of the methotrexate; laxatives to counteract the side-effects of the opioids; supplements to replenish potassium depletion.

Your pain has significantly eased in the last few days. You've slowly begun eating again. You've managed to walk round your hospital room without using the drip stand to support you.

And now you're coming home for a night, you start to feel pretty good.

A glimmer of optimism takes hold of you as your dad helps you from the car and you're greeted by your mum and sister.

This scene is jittery and nervous but content. Hopeful. Maybe things will be okay.

At home you climb into your own bed and revel in the familiar textures and smells. The comfort.

You open your window and breathe clean, fresh air. It feels almost foreign. It fills your nose and throat and lungs and you smile a wide, involuntary smile.

Downstairs you take a pint glass and fill it to the brim with fresh, cold water. Today there's no tiny cups and lukewarm water from plastic jugs. The tap water is cool, clear and infinitely refreshing. You had no idea how much you missed it. You glug it down noisily, almost desperately, letting it spill clumsily over your chin and onto your chest. You finish the glass and place it down on the kitchen side. Again, you grin to yourself, and drag your heavy legs back upstairs.

It's evening and you're sat with your family watching TV. They drink cups of tea and eat the same chocolate biscuits they always used to. You sip a nutrient shake unenthusiastically.

Your sister glances at you every few minutes and you catch her eye, smiling each time.

Before long you find yourself drifting away to sleep and your mum helps you upstairs to bed. She says goodnight and you're alone. The large plastic bag of medicine is sat on the bedside table beside you. You consider your pain: a fuzzy headache but not much more. Nevertheless, you convince yourself it's for the best to take some codeine anyway. Away from the stare of the nurses, you take three pills – 90mg, not 60mg as prescribed.

What follows is a serene, dreamless sleep.

You wake up late in the morning. A night's rest without observations has been gloriously peaceful.

Looking at your bed, you see that the sheets are scattered with endless flakes of dead skin. You try to brush it all to the floor but it's an impossible operation. For some reason you feel too embarrassed to tell your mum.

Soon enough it's time to go back to hospital. Nobody makes a fuss of this. You wave to your mum and sister. They wave back. The drive is long and your dad is silent for almost all of it. Songs call out from the radio, each lyric seeming like a plea.

Once you arrive, things quickly fall into routine. You change back into pyjamas and climb into bed. A nurse comes and takes your obs. Tubes are attached to your Hickman line. You hug your dad, wires and tubes separating you, and say goodbye.

And then, again, you're alone.

You look out of your window and see your dad walking alone across the car park. He looks the same as anyone else out there; just a man going about his business. He settles into the front seat of his car and closes the door. And he just sits. He sits for what seems like an hour. You're transfixed. Eventually, almost reluctantly, his car creeps slowly from the car park and disappears towards the exit.

Later in the evening, your consultant comes to visit. He checks that everything went okay at home. He explains that tonight they will start you on your second cycle of chemotherapy.

'There'll be some similar challenges to the first cycle, but there might be new things to deal with too – we'll just watch out for those and keep an eye on your progress.'

And then, just as he's leaving, almost as if he's read your mind, he adds: 'We won't know how well the disease has or hasn't responded to treatment until the results of the scans, which will be after cycle four. So just sit tight.'

He gathers his clipboard and a few sheets of paper and then goes.

Out of your window, faint brushstrokes of orange and red are bleeding through the clouds as the sun sets and the world outside begins to pack itself away.

The scene in your room is all ticks and beeps and clicks and drips.

You think painfully of home.

A nurse wakes you. It's dark outside. She connects the first bag of the new cycle of chemotherapy. You look at it indifferently. The nurse asks if you're okay. You tell her yes but your head hurts. She fetches 60mg of codeine for you. You swallow them with lukewarm water. She pats you on the shoulder and you turn over and sleep.

Shapes move lazily before your eyes.

There is golden light, cast coolly on the floor, and the air is dense with murmurs and whispers.

You feel detached.

You hear voices fade in and out of focus.

Phrases, half-constructed: 'lack of response… continued mediastinal growth… irregular patterns… suspected hypermetabolic… depletion prevents further… options limited.'

Your consultant shakes you gently into the room. His eyes twinkle with care and sadness.

Behind him stand your family. And your friends.

Nobody is crying.

They're bathed in light.

Their smiles speak of nothing but love.

You awake from the dream. It's the darkest hour of the night and the ward feels eerie.

The scene is cold.

Your dream haunts the room. You wear it like a blanket. The warmth in the faces of your family and friends comforts you.

You begin to consider, and perhaps for the first time to

believe, that this treatment might not work, and that soon you might die.

And to your own surprise, this is okay.

All life, you realise, is chance. Birth is a game of numbers. Disease and death are the same. Numbers and chance determine who lives and who dies. And if the odds are against you here, there's no fighting it. There's no dignity in complaining. No rationality in lamenting your luck. Numbers are not partial; they do not care for who you are or what you want to be.

You sit up in your bed, alone as ever, and do what seems like the natural thing: you begin to plan your funeral.

On a scrappy notebook you scribble down all the important details.

You choose music that you love.

You select quotations that seem apt.

You think about your friends and your family.

You fight back tears and pen a message to those you'll leave behind.

And when it's done, you look at the notes and you listen to the stillness of the ward, and you imagine in your head and then see before you those smiling faces, and you hear the songs you've chosen rising high to the ceiling, and you see that the scene is drenched in colour – amber and gold – and a calm and content glow reflects in the eyes of everyone there, and you cannot help but smile, and you think that maybe, just maybe, it's all for the best.

I'm sorry, I can't help you.

Since you returned to hospital to begin your second cycle of chemotherapy, there has been a noise in your room. It's a strange, troubling sound. A kind of screeching noise. Somewhere between mechanical and electric.

Alone in your bed at night, the noise fills your head.

The next round of chemo is starting to hit you. Once again, your head twinges and throbs and your guts burn.

Your second and third intrathecal injections have been almost as disastrous as the first: you think back to them at night, your palms clammy with sweat, ghostly jolts twitching down your spine.

The pain is again making it difficult to walk. The nurses have started to bring you cardboard water bottles just like before, to save you the struggle of leaving your bed in the night to urinate. The sight of them fills you with shame.

You creep to the bathroom one morning to attempt to wash yourself. As you walk, you lean heavily on your drip stand for support. You allow yourself a long glance in the mirror and the reflection looking back at you fills you with abject pity.

Those spiritless eyes. Blackened scabs on the lips. The awful patches of peeling skin on the face and neck. The terrible, raw, burning rash on the arms and legs. You realise now that even your eyebrows and eyelashes have gone. The effect is terrifying: you look barely human.

When visitors come, you ask them about the noise. But during the day it seems quieter or at least less noticeable over the humdrum of daytime hospital business. One of the registrars seems concerned by your obsession with it.

'Try to forget about it. Perhaps you should wear earplugs at night,' he suggests.

'I do,' you protest, 'but I can still hear it.'

He looks at you almost sternly. 'I'm sorry, I can't help you. I'll ask the nursing staff to investigate.'

In the bleak, dim evenings and the terrible, long, painful nights, you are consumed by two things: pain and noise. As the fire burns grimly through your guts, the screeching escalates inside your head, each tearing at the edges of your brain.

Pain and noise.

'Make it stop,' you plead to no-one.

You cringe and sweat.

You flinch at the air.

They prescribe heroin again.

The diamorphine pump is wheeled in; the silver trolley with the enormous syringe housed in the bright blue casing; activated by key only. In the darkness, numbers flash up on the little screen and you yearn for the pain to melt away. You plead for sleep.

All the while the screeching noise stops and starts, the soundtrack to your torment.

You shiver with pain.

The pain nurse administers additional morphine via intramuscular injection to your stomach.

'Can you hear that noise?' you ask. 'How do I stop it?'

'I'm sorry,' she says, 'I can't help you.'

In the darkest hour of the night, there is no noise on the ward. Nothing but the screeching sound in your room and the slow, heavy rise and fall of your breath.

Morphine takes hold of your dreams. The darkness seems huge and cruel, almost endless.

Figures loom over you with silent menace.

Eyes hang demonically above your head.

The room around you seems to twist as you jerk in and out of consciousness.

You're a little boy, being chased through the fields near your childhood home.

There's a man standing in your hospital room, his face masked by shadow.

You're swimming in the sea and you lose control; a wave pulls you under and you panic and your mother is screaming.

There is a man in your hospital room. He looks down at you. Expressionless. His eyes are huge and they pierce right into you. You're afraid.

You're at a park. A storm is coming. You're alone. Enormous black clouds swell ominously above. This is what terror feels like.

There is a man in your room who wants to kill you. He will kill you. This is what terror feels like.

A deafening otherworldly noise fills the room, screeching at you, bouncing off the walls of your skull, and death itself hangs above you grinning with manic glee.

This is what terror feels like.

Somewhere, someone screams.

The night slips quietly into morning and the thin, pale light rouses you from your rest. The dreams have ended. Your bed is damp with sweat.

There are imprints on your arms and side from where you've slept on the wires from your Hickman line. They've become tangled and blood has backed up into the tubes.

This scene feels dense and thick.

Around your room, assorted medical equipment stands idly, watchfully: an observation trolley with its endless wires; an oxygen mask and ruffled hose connected to a canister; a drip stand with its empty bag hanging limply depleted; the diamorphine pump encased in blue plastic clamped onto its silver trolley – a constant, bleak reminder of where you are.

And all the while, scarcely ceasing, intermittent but interminable, is the mind-bending screech and click and buzz of that noise in your room, spitting at you in the stillness of the morning, welcoming you to a new day.

Your friends are here. So is a nurse. Or a doctor. Someone is attaching something to you. Or removing it.

You squint at the faces around you. Someone is talking. You feel like there's a thousand eyes on you. Someone takes your hand and holds it. This scene feels familiar. Like déjà vu. You laugh.

You awake and it's late. You're alone. The ward is asleep. You feel quite lucid.

Checking the morphine pump, you realise the nurse has reduced the dosage. You can feel pain in your head, your legs, your guts and your back, but it's manageable. You drink some water and it tastes artificial, as ever.

Looking round your room, you see the cards people have sent you and the gifts – they give you strength.

You try to work out how far through the treatment you are but you realise you have no idea what day it is. Your phone is out of battery.

Soon, the peace of the night is broken, maddeningly, by the scratching noise in your room. But this time there is no anger or annoyance; instead you feel something closer to resilience.

You move your arms into a position to force your body upright. This takes longer than you imagined; your muscles are stiff and weak. Sat, propped up by pillows, you reach forward and drag the baby-blue NHS blanket from your bed to reveal your legs. They look wasted. The skin is yellow wherever it isn't flaming red.

With almost reverent care, you lean forward and take one of your legs, lift it up, swing it round, and let it drop gently to the ground. The cold, cool surface of the floor feels strange. You gingerly do the same with your other leg and let it drop. Now you are sat with both feet touching the floor. Your heart is racing and your breathing is fast.

Holding the drip stand for support, you very slowly attempt to raise yourself from your bed and into an upright position. But as soon as you're standing, your knee buckles and you slump back onto the bed, panting.

You consider giving up.

You consider throwing your drip stand across the room, watching the bag of chemo splatter against the wall and the morphine pump smash open on the ground. You picture the Hickman line being ripped from your chest. But you know you don't have the strength to do this.

The noise scratches and squeaks, reverberating off the walls.

Locking your knees tightly in place, you stand up again and push your weight down onto the heavy drip stand. You wobble, but this time you remain upright.

You smile to yourself.

For days you have been convinced that this noise must be coming from one of the medical instruments that line the perimeter of your room. All those dials and buttons and displays.

With significant caution, you begin to wheel yourself towards the edge of the room, guided as much by the noise as you are by what you can see through the darkness.

You press your ear to the walls and listen intently, moving

just a few inches at a time, trying to locate the sound.

It takes you what feels like an hour to navigate the full perimeter of the room, checking every single possible object, whether suspicious or innocent.

At no point when it sounds does the noise seem any louder or any quieter.

Finally, you return to your bed – bemused and exhausted and aching and angry.

As you are about to give up, close to defeat, the noise screams out at you again in the moonlight. Louder this time than before, you're sure of it. Much louder than when you were on the opposite side of the room.

You survey the objects directly above and around your bed carefully, but none are responsible. It sounds out again, almost mockingly.

And it is then that something strikes you, like an epiphany: your bed itself is mechanical. It has an electronic control pad which adjusts the height and angle.

Adrenaline rushes through your body. You consider calling for a nurse, but you know they can't help you. Not with this. Delicately, you lower yourself down onto one knee, and tentatively push an ear towards the space underneath the bed.

You wait.

This wait feels like an eternity.

Sweat pours down your neck and back.

At last, you hear it, louder and more brutal than you've ever heard it: the noise is coming from under your bed.

Blood throbs in your ears. Your heart thumps against your ribs. You lower yourself onto both knees, and then with tremendous effort use your aching arms to push yourself onto the floor so you're lying flat on your stomach.

The wires from the chemo and the morphine snake down from the drip stand into the Hickman line in your chest, and both tubes are now pressed against the cold, hard floor of your hospital room.

Using your arms to push yourself along the floor, like some bizarre swimming stroke, you maneuver yourself underneath the bed and with one, final ounce of strength you roll over onto your back so you're lying facing upwards.

The solution is startlingly simple. Almost frustratingly so. A plug has come loose, the one connecting the mechanism which operates the bed to the electric supply.

Just as you go to push it in, the noise screams out at you for one final time, like a dying bird, and you silence it with an infinitely satisfying click of plastic into place.

Stillness and sanity surround you.

As you triumphantly but cautiously drag yourself out from under the bed and, using the drip stand for support, back into an upright position, a whole world of relief washes over you and you privately rank this success as perhaps your life's greatest achievement.

You turn around, slide your legs back between the sheets, and collapse onto your pillow with a jubilant smile plastered across your face.

You grin and you laugh and you absorb the peaceful silence and the solitude of the ward.

And when you sleep it is perhaps the calmest and most beautiful sleep you have ever had, or ever will.

You're half way there.

There's a cricket pitch on the other side of the hospital car park that you can see from your room. This morning there's a man out there mowing the grass.

A bird flies soundlessly past your window.

There are little white buds on the branches of the trees.

This scene is all delicate hints of warmth and springtime cliché.

You can't hear the outside world, but you imagine the sound of the mower buzzing hungrily through the grass.

You've been given a few days for your body to recover from the second cycle of chemo and soon you will start your third. You feel calm and determined.

You eat some food: half a bowl of soup – cream of chicken – followed by a nutritional milkshake.

Somebody else has been bringing your food this week, a man. He's also bright and cheerful.

He calls you 'champ.'

Sunshine threatens the view from your window with warmth. You yearn to step outside, and slowly begin to dress yourself in anticipation with fresh pyjamas, a dressing gown and slippers.

The morning is drawing to a close and you become agitated. You want the nurse to take your obs as soon as possible so you can step outside and breathe the fresh air.

You can see blossom on the breeze and you ache to be outside. You stand obsessively by the window, watching.

After a while, a man and a woman amble out from the

entrance downstairs, followed by a nurse.

Both patients are bald and ageless and wear droopy dressing gowns. Each has a white surgical mask covering the mouth and nose. Their facial expressions are hidden.

Eventually, a nurse comes in and takes your observations. She makes her notes and goes to leave.

'Can I go outside for a minute?' you ask. 'I just really fancy some fresh air.'

She smiles at you sadly. 'No I'm sorry darling, not today. Your levels are too low. There's too much of an infection risk. Maybe in the next couple of days.'

Disappointment hangs in the air long after she's gone.

In this room everything is sterile – from the sheets on which you sleep, to the water that you drink, to their air that you breathe – it's how it has to be, you know that, but it feels so cold and unnatural.

You turn to the window and watch as the two bald patients stand rigidly in the fresh wind. After a while, they slope back inside.

Your mum and dad come to visit, arriving early in the morning. It's been three days since the weather began to change and people from the ward downstairs have been allowed to walk outside. The doctors have yet to allow you to step out from your ward.

It's not even 9am when your dad practically bounces into the room.

'Fancy a day at home?' He grins widely.

'Seriously?'

'Doctors say you can have twenty-four hours,' adds your mum. 'Let's get you ready!'

You walk through the ward to the lift, flanked by your parents. The doctors make you wear a surgical mask while you're outside but you can take it off once you're indoors.

A nurse pushes a giant yellow box on wheels labeled 'CYTOTOXIC WASTE' and joins the three of you heading downstairs.

There are no mirrors in the lift.

As you gingerly make your way to the exit, you notice the nurse park the yellow box next to three others – green, red and black. From here you can't read what these boxes say.

Stepping out through the doors of the ward and into the car park is an anticlimax. It's colder than you imagined, and the surgical mask makes it difficult to breathe.

It seems almost impossibly noisy outside. Bizarrely, and just momentarily, you feel an urge to turn around and return to the security and familiarity of your room on the ward.

The scene is uncomfortable.

You're grateful when you reach the car and the door closes with a comforting click.

On the journey home you sleep. You're still wearing pyjamas and a dressing gown, but you've optimistically packed proper clothes. Nestled in your lap is the NHS-branded plastic bag filled with all your drugs. It's even fuller than last time. You've lost track of what you're taking, but there's a green sheet inside on which, hand-written, is a complicated looking matrix of drug names and times of the day. As the nurse put this into the bag, you made a quiet decision to delegate this responsibility to your mum.

You awake just as the car reaches your home town. It seems to ghost silently through the busy streets that teem with everyday life.

Waking up in the car, just as you reach home, reminds

you of returning from holidays as a child. You remember yourself hunched over like this in the back of your dad's car, tiny and weary and sleepy.

Both parents help you from the car into the house and you settle onto the sofa to rest. Your mum fusses with your bag of medication, which when handled by someone else seems implausibly large – do you really need to take all these pills every day? You find your eyes covertly scanning for the painkillers, and you relax when you see there's both codeine and oramorph.

Your dad brings you a cup of tea.

'So,' he says. 'How'd you like to surprise your grand-parents?'

It's your grandparents' anniversary weekend and your dad has hatched a plan to surprise them with a visit. They're expecting your mum, dad and sister, but have no idea you'll be there.

Your dad asks you to wait for a moment while he goes up to tell them he has an anniversary surprise.

You begin walking up the gravel to their house, holding in your hand the balloon your dad has bought. You're wearing a white surgical mask. Your mum and sister walk behind.

Your grandparents are elderly and have been unable to make it to the hospital to see you.

They have yet to see you since you began treatment.

They have yet to see you frail and bald.

Urged on by your dad, your grandmother walks down the gravel path and stops in her tracks the moment she sees you. She brings her hand up to her mouth and her face instantly contorts. Tears stream from her eyes.

When she reaches you, she grips you tightly. She says nothing.

You and your family stay with your grandparents in their living room for around an hour.

This scene is caring and jovial.

On the mantelpiece is a photograph of you and your sister from your childhood. You're sat on a beach with your arm around her. You both smile proudly, showcasing your sandcastles. Next to it is another photograph, this time of you at university, just last year. Your photograph smiles back at you broadly, well-fed and comfortable and with a full head of hair. It's strange to feel jealous of yourself.

Eventually you begin to tire and your mum suggests taking you home. You hug both your grandparents in turn but as you do, a tantalising and terrible thought takes hold of you: if this treatment doesn't work, this may be the last time you ever seen them. Icy water trickles through you.

As you walk back down the gravel path to the car, you turn and look at your grandparents' house.

You think of Christmas food and your grandmother's cakes. Watching your grandfather work on crosswords. Summer afternoons in their garden with your sister.

Memories flood through you. They flash by.

Through the translucent veil of the glass door, now some distance away, you can just make out your grandparents, still stood there, holding each other in a long embrace.

It's overcast when your dad takes you back to the hospital in his car.

There are two men debating politics on the radio. The argument is heated and they talk over each other. You can hear the intakes of breath from each as they move to interject.

Words fall from them in cascades. Sound bites.

Responsibility.

Doing the right thing.

Time to act.

Grown-up decisions.

Your dad leans over and turns the radio off.

When you first made this journey, two months ago, the car was full of people and possessions, and tension and adrenaline seemed to pulse through the air.

Your dad used a SatNav because he didn't know the way.

Now he knows the route by heart.

Today the car is empty except for you, your dad, and your overnight bag.

As you walk onto the ward, two doctors sprint past you into a room across the hall, a room just like yours. They disappear into silence. Your dad places his hand on your back and steers you away.

Darkness has fallen outside and your room is softly lit. It feels cosy. You're tired and you feel almost relieved to be back. This feeling sits uncomfortably with you. You swallow the guilt.

Your dad gives you a bear hug and you suddenly feel a wave of sorrow for him.

You think about the long journey home in the dark with the mindless, meaningless noise of the radio the only distraction from his thoughts. You think about the number of times he's had to do this journey already, often alone, and the thoughts that must occupy his head every time. You wonder, does he think to himself, 'Will I ever see my son again?'

When he lets you go, your dad looks you straight in the eye.

'You're half way there,' he says, robustly.

You try to smile. 'I know.'

'Half way there,' he repeats, and he squeezes your shoulder as he turns to leave. 'Remember. Call us any time. For anything.'

'I will. Thank you.'

He smiles at the ground and closes the door softly behind him.

This time you're too tired and it's probably too dark to watch him out the window, but you imagine his walk to the car and the journey home and the thoughts that must haunt him. You wish there was someone who could tell him everything was going to be okay, like he told you in the kitchen on the day of your diagnosis.

As you lie in bed in the dim light, in your mind you picture – from an enormous height – the tiny light of his car moving through the darkness, winding along the motorway back home, like a nerve signal down a spine, speeding away from you, moving between worlds, carrying with it whatever hope, and strength, he has left.

It passes the time.

There's strength in your legs today so you venture out from your room and onto the ward. You shuffle to a vending machine down the hall.

A boy is wheeled in by a nurse, his eyes wide. He looks young, maybe late teens. A girl hangs by his elbow. She's younger, maybe his sister. A very tired, grey man follows them.

The boy steps out from his chair and his frame seems to slump under its own weight. He approaches the counter and talks quietly to a nurse. She tells him to sit back down, and he does.

After a while he sees you staring. Your gut flinches.

He gestures. You walk over. Introductions are exchanged. Weak handshakes.

He has leukaemia. Sometime it's okay, sometime it's bad, he says. His eyebrows arch – he's never met anyone with lymphoma before. Nobody as young as you anyway.

'How long have you been in treatment?' you ask.

'Two years,' he says.

He's cheerful.

His hair is short but he's not bald. You wonder how quickly hair grows back between treatments.

'So what chemo are you on?' you ask.

He explains his regimen. You've heard of some of the drugs, but not all. The schedule is different. He'll be here for two weeks, maybe three, then he'll be going home for a while.

He asks you about your chemo and you explain.

The boy looks at you earnestly. 'So. How do you feel?'

His father and his sister shift uncomfortably. They don't make eye contact with you. The nurse is talking to a colleague at the counter.

'Okay today,' you say. 'But some days I can't walk. And the drugs make me feel spaced-out.' You find yourself smiling. 'I wish I could go outside.'

The boy smiles back. 'Yeah, doesn't everyone?'

There's a pause. 'You got a console?' he asks.

'Yeah. But it gives me headaches. So does the TV.'

'Oh… that's a shame. It passes the time.'

'Yeah?'

'Yeah,' he says. 'That's what it's all about really, in here. How to pass the time.'

'Sounds like prison.'

He laughs.

You both look at the ground.

The scene feels awkward.

You make your excuses and you leave.

You used to read. You used to watch TV and films. You used to listen to music. You used to write. You used to fantasise about travelling, about hiking through hills and crossing the ocean.

Now you wish only for sleep.

You take painkillers.

It passes the time.

Daytime TV. Nightmares. Infusions of chemotherapy into your blood. Injections of chemotherapy into your spine. Blood falls from your mouth into a cup.

This is your third cycle of chemo.

You run your fingers over your ribs. Before you became ill, you were overweight. You ate too much and drank too much. Your face was round and your cheeks flushed red when you laughed.

Now the bones in your forearm make you feel like a cheap

Halloween costume. Your eyes bulge in hollow sockets.

Dietitians see you regularly. The milkshakes they prescribe taste increasingly worse. You have no appetite. Once again, you dismiss eating entirely. Everything you drink burns your throat. You take on fluid through a drip.

Things don't seem to matter much to you anymore.

Your daily puzzle is how best to ride the next wave of discomfort. It's frustrating to have neither the energy nor the inclination to take interest in the things you used to. You feel pathetic and one-dimensional. You take as many painkillers as they will give you. It passes the time.

Your consultant comes to see you. He's wearing a polythene apron and rubber gloves and a mask. He tells you that your immune system is very, very weak at the moment.

'So. How do you feel?' he asks.

You say nothing for a while, as you build up some saliva in your mouth. 'My throat hurts. So does my stomach.'

He looks at you for a few long seconds. You feel your eyes rolling. He leaves.

Soon after he's gone, a nurse comes in with some oramorph and she feeds you two spoonfuls of the syrup, straight into your mouth like you're a child. You swallow, with trouble. Your mind slips into a pleasant, foggy, half-sleep.

Birds fly past your window. They soar and dive. Outside your door, men and women in white coats dash by in a blur.

Alone, you picture your bed drifting on a boundless blue sea, the waves rising and falling with your breath.

Your room smells like the old swimming pool your dad used to take you to as a kid, to pass the time on Saturday mornings.

There's a show on TV about children in hospitals. A celebrity is visiting a little girl with cancer. Her room is full of teddy bears and colourful toys. There's an oxygen tube under her nose and a two wires attached to her forearm. A drip stands silently in the background. Her bed sheets are the same as yours – blue on white. She wears a pink and yellow bandana on her head.

They interview the girl's mother. She says her daughter never complains. Always smiling.

The celebrity is moved to tears. Such strength. Such noble spirit.

You lie in bed and feel nothing but shame. Your legs are weak and yellow. There are cardboard bottles of urine on the floor. Your sheets are full of dead skin and dried blood. Your head throbs and you ache. Deep inside you is a feeling of disgrace and disgust – you think of that little girl, smiling through her pain.

Through your door's window you can see the boy with leukaemia you spoke to a few days ago. He's talking to a nurse out on the ward. They laugh.

Shame turns to resentment as you realise just how alone you really are.

It's a dull and sober day on the ward and some friends are due to visit.

When you wake you feel sick, and the feeling only gets worse as the morning goes on. You send a text to cancel. You need to sleep. When your friend responds, he seems disappointed but says they all understand and wish you well. They miss you. You say you miss them too. But if you're honest with yourself, you know that isn't true.

Cancer has changed you, and the person you are now would have nothing to say to your friends. You barely have anything to say to your family. Maybe you can go back to who you used to be, but for now you feel like you're someone else, watching yourself from without.

You awake in the night with a feeling in your gut like a cork-screw turning. You double up, bringing your knees to your mouth and you gnaw at the skin. The pain rises from your abdomen up into your chest and you gasp. You cry out – it's a pathetic noise, like an distressed animal. You feel abused. You feel your pulse in your head. There's poison in your body.

The dark brown pouch hangs on the drip stand, ominous in the silence of the night. You press the button that calls for the nurse. She asks what you need and you can barely speak. She shines a torch into your face and then hurries away.

When she returns, someone else is with her. You close your eyes tightly and struggle against the will to moan as the pain rises through your guts in waves. One of the nurses places a hand on your head and feeds you a spoonful of oramorph. You shiver. After a while someone leaves and returns with a third person. You hear them talking but can't follow the conversation. Just odd words. *Convulsions. Damp with sweat. Can't focus.*

The third person calls your name and you see a face flash quickly in front of you, and then it's gone.

Your stomach burns and you feel yourself retching.

They ask you to lie still. There's a sharp sting in your belly as someone administers an intramuscular injection.

Voices fade.

The scene is suddenly bird's eye view. There's a boy in a bed, a skeleton, surrounded by medical staff, blood and vomit on his sheets, his limbs twisted and his face contorted. As the morphine flows through him he softens, relaxes, and, as he finally exhales deeply, so does the scene.

The next day you feel numb and frail and your insides burn.
    You lift your arm to look at your phone. The image blurs.
    People in coats come to read numbers on dials.
    Nobody smiles.

As the pain abates, you are dealt a new blow: you have a bowel infection. The doctor says it's called 'c. difficile' and it's a dangerous infection so they'll need to monitor you closely.

You barely have the strength to lift yourself out of bed but you must do so every few minutes, to sit sadly and pathetically on the cold toilet seat in the bathroom. The cramps in your stomach suggest vomit and diarrhoea.

The infection makes you sweat more than ever.

It's days before the discomfort softens. In the night, you stare, wide-eyed, into the darkness.

Your sister comes to visit. She is sat in the blue vinyl chair in your room. She's come up on the train to visit you. She rests her hands on a cushion on her lap.

There's a box of chocolates on the top of a pile by her feet.

'Who are these from?' she asks.

'I don't know...'

She looks at them more closely. 'Are you gonna eat them?'

'No.'

'Can I?'

'You want to eat my cancer chocolates?'

'Well if you're not going to...'

You find yourself smiling. 'Go ahead.'

As the minutes pass, few words are exchanged between you, but the scene is comfortable. Almost cosy. You breathe heavily.

'So the nurses said you're on antibiotics?'

You gesture to the drip. There's a large, clear fluid bag and a smaller bag containing off-yellow antibiotics. 'Yeah. Seems to be working okay. I'm in much less pain. Still need to go to the toilet a lot though.'

'Yeah...'

'In fact...' You push yourself up into a sitting position and delicately swing your legs out of your bed. Using the drip stand for support, you edge slowly to your bathroom. Your sister has been with you for less than an hour when you have to do this for the third time. By then she's eaten most of your chocolates.

When you mention this she smiles broadly and you find yourself laughing with her. It's a warm, safe feeling.

Finally, when it's time for her to go, you hug for a long time. You look at her closely and try to figure out if she's okay. Her eyes are dry. Her voice doesn't shake as she says goodbye. She seems so strong. You want to tell her that it's okay, that she doesn't need to pretend, that she can cry if she wants to. Maybe it would help. Or maybe she doesn't need to. Maybe she has the strength of the little girl from the TV show. And suddenly in that moment your sister is your hero. As she leaves your room and walks through the ward, back to her own world, her big brother sat trembling alone in a hospital bed, she seems to you to be stronger than anyone you've ever met.

The antibiotics control the worst of the infection, and the painkillers seem to help, but you still find yourself sat on the toilet every few minutes. Each night is an endless cruel joke: as soon as your drowsy eyes close and you slip into slumber, your gut twists and your bowel contorts and you wearily trudge back to the bathroom. Soon enough, you give up much hope of sleeping, and you turn on the TV and through the fog of the morphine you watch the colours dance on the screen. It passes the time.

'How many times did you open your bowels last night?' your consultant asks.

'Maybe five times.'

'Good. Much better. You're improving. You must be fighting the infection. We'll do another two days of antibiotics and then see where we are.'

'Okay.'

'How's the pain?'

You think about the little girl on the TV show.

You think about the other boy on the ward.

You think about your sister.

'It's okay,' you say. 'It's getting better.'

'Great. Then we'll take you off the morphine for now and see how that goes.' He smiles. 'You're doing okay, you know.'

That night, as the morphine wears off, the pain in your guts feels like fire. You try to ignore it but you can't.

When you eventually call for the nurse, the sweat has soaked through your pyjamas to the sheets.

The oramorph helps you relax, and after a while the pain subsides.

You trudge to and from the bathroom throughout the night. Stood in front of the mirror, staring sadly into your own eyes, you see only weakness. You feel only shame.

It's your choice.

Keep walking.

You're outside your body.

Talking to yourself in second person.

This hill you can climb. You can. Keep going. Just keep walking.

You're thin and you're bald and you're probably dying and the heat hits you like a car.

Sweat drips.

Your body aches with poisonous, sinister fire.

You look down at your feet, watch them move as if in slow motion. The hill climbs.

Above there are clouds and you try to remember the last time you walked anywhere unaccompanied.

When did you last put your feet up and watch TV?

When did you last read a book?

Now ask yourself: 'Why are you walking?'

There's a crossroads. Left, right, or straight on. Behind you is the hospital.

You take the left.

Go back a few minutes.

You're in the car park. Your hands are clammy.

Around you is so much noise. Your head throbs. Air fills your nostrils like water. An old couple shuffle towards a car and it beeps and the lights flash on and off.

You squint.

A man, maybe in his thirties, pushes a wheelchair. A little girl sits inside it, still. She's bald. There are tubes falling out of her nose and arm. Fabric patterned with flowers. There's mucus on her face. Blood on her lips. Her eyes are open. They're yellow.

You watch the man as he trundles towards the ward. In the wind he twitches.

Go back a few hours.

You've finished your third cycle of chemo, the pain is falling away and you've been disconnected from your fluid drip. Your consultant is happy with your blood levels. The nurse says you can go outside.

'How long for?' you ask.

'It's your choice,' she says.

Outside is a world of unknowable possibility. The hospital smell seems suddenly suffocating; sterile, like chlorine in your lungs.

Go forward a few weeks.

You're choking and trying to shout out. There's blood on your pillow and on your bed sheets.

Back in the car park, an insect dances above you.

Sunlight briefly pierces the clouds.

The tarmac smells like bonfires and you think of your early teens. Burning plastic and wood and metal.

The grass looks too green to be real.

Noises compete.

This scene is all yawning metal and the rumble of conversation and the distant tune of sirens.

You reach the main road. Cars fly past at improbable speed, and you shake.

Go back to that night on the balcony.

You coughed so violently. You felt so sad.

Did you know then? Could you have?

Back to the hill.

You swing your body round to look at how far you've come and the road seems to stretch for miles. The hospital is small in the distance, masked by trees. You hold your thumb up in front of your eye and behind it the hospital disappears.

Like it was never there.

The hill gets steeper the higher you climb. Your breath gets caught in your chest. You splutter and stumble but it's just one foot after another.

The thrill of the fresh air and forgotten smells and the novelty of activity have subsided and what's left is just the monotony of the motion of your legs. A determination to climb.

This is your Everest.

Go forward a few years.

Whiskey and beer. You try to catch memories, like butterflies. You thrash and turn in the night. Grope through darkness. Music on your laptop. Beeps and clicks. Dim light.

Can you remember how it felt?

You're at the top of the hill. The climb has made you weaker than you expected.

You lurch into a chip shop.

Eyes follow you.

You're bald and you're stumbling.

Underneath your shirt is your Hickman line, that impossible tube that hangs from your chest.

In your blood flow codeine and chemo and cancer.

Place your order.

Eat.

This might be the last time you get to eat food like this.

The idea hangs in the air above you. It lingers. You smell the vinegar on your fingers and the salt feels coarse, like sand.

You're a child on the beach. On holiday.

You warily walk from the chip shop to the pub across the road and when you enter, nobody looks at you.

The pub is cold and dingy.

This scene is all fruit machines and groups of men squatting on stools around dark wooden tables.

There's football on a big screen, and all the men are pointed towards it. You approach the bar.

'What will it be?'

You cast your eyes over the beers. The labels blur. Your words slur. 'What do you recommend?'

'It's your choice.'

You buy your drink and sit down to watch the match.

Colours and movement.

Muttering, chattering, shouting.

The wooden table sticks to the skin on your wrist.

On the menu, the ink has blotched and blurred; the words are unclear.

Beer tastes alien to you.

Men call out to each other and slap each other's backs.

Colours merge.

You're alone.

Slowly you rise from your table and you leave.

Outside the pub, sunlight whitens the air.

Nobody knows where you are. The walk back to the hospital is long and tiring but you find yourself smiling.

This is your secret.

You see a bus stop. You could get on a bus and go anywhere you want. You could leave the hospital and nobody would know where you'd gone.

Your room awaits. Chemo and painkillers.

It's your choice.

Go forward a few years.
  You're a long way from home. You're alone. You cough.

Back in the car park and the air feels thin. The sky looks strange, almost fickle. Your legs are even heavier than usual. There are fewer cars. Where before there was urgency, the paced has slowed. People are heading home.

Your hands run unconsciously over the scars on your neck and chest.

The hospital corridors remain alive with activity. Trolleys roll past you, all part of the organic dance of daily movement. Some carry food; others carry people.
  You stand at the entrance to the ward and you breathe in.
  The doors open, and the silence breaks.

You're doing so well.

The needle touches a nerve in your back. You wince. The pillow between your knees is drenched with sweat. Déjà vu. The doctor exhales and clicks his tongue in frustration and the nurse's hand soothingly rubs your shoulder.

Your friends come to visit. You sit up in bed, feeling meek and tired but stronger than you have in a while.

This cycle of chemo, your fourth, your last of the regimen, seems to be going much better than the previous three. The pain has been manageable. You've avoided infection.

'You're doing so well,' they say.

Optimism creeps into your voice as you laugh with your friends. They sit around your bed in a semi-circle.

This scene is all newspaper clippings and apple juice and chocolate muffins and relieved smiles.

Headaches are background noise; the throb is a ticking clock.

Concentrate on conversation.

Drugs move through you, just part of your daily diet. You no longer check to see what you're taking or why.

Your appetite is improving. You delicately feed yourself a tuna and cucumber sandwich from its blue and white cardboard box. After that it's carrot soup with two blue and white packets of salt.

This is the fourth month of your stay in hospital. It feels like longer. You struggle to remember how you felt before you came here.

That you is a different you.

At night you willfully lose yourself in the thud and pump

and colour of the TV. Late-night laughter tumbles from the screen and out into the blue-lit room. It dances down the corridors and into the ward.

Numb boredom eats at you. Your attention is weak; your head twinges when you focus too hard. Your mind wanders between dreams and fantasies.

As you fight for lucidity, the tension and uncertainty surfaces within you and you pine for the sedate listlessness of opiates.

Without pain, you are lost.

You're in limbo, stuck in a world between nightmare and grim reality.

You miss home.

Only in the darkest hours of the night do you admit to yourself the possibility that this soon might all be over; that they'll let you go home, to be with your family.

You count the days.

Time seems to drift past you like fog.

You sleep on your back, and as you drift away your fingers now routinely caress the Hickman line in your chest. From the drip bag it carries the tonic that may cure you or kill you.

It is what binds you to your future, if you have one.

It nourishes and assaults you, like some grotesque umbilical cord.

When your parents come to visit, you struggle. You have to sleep. They're chipper. You apologise.

'You've been through so much,' your mum says, her voice full of optimism and kindness. 'And you're so close to the end! You're doing so well.'

So close to the end.

So close to the end.

Your dad says something but you don't hear. His voice fades into a murmur. When your eyes open, they've gone.

Each night you shift from nightmare to nightmare.

Machines beep and click.

There's pain in your chest – tightness, and a sting when you breathe in.

Doctors are concerned. A registrar comes to do a physical exam.

Your eyes dart.

Breathe in and hold your breath.

Breathe normally.

Repeat.

The registrar looks at you. He seems worried.

'I think you might have an infection.' He goes to make a call.

Pretty soon he's back, followed by a man wheeling an enormous trolley that barely makes its way through the door. They're both wearing masks and polythene gloves. Together they unfold a cumbersome plastic arm and position it over your bed.

'We're going to take an X-Ray,' the registrar says. 'But we need to keep you here.'

They set up the X-Ray machine, switch off the lights, leave the room, come back, then turn the lights on again. They do this twice.

As the equipment is wheeled away, the registrar calls back to you, his voice muffled through his mask. 'You're doing well!'

Heat. Sweat. Dry mouth. Discomfort.

Something flares inside you. You fidget. The antibiotics

sit above you, dripping steadily. They don't seem to have worked, at least not yet. You can feel the now familiar slow bubble of infection stirring in your gut. Every few minutes the cramps make you shudder.

Hopelessly you press the button to call for help.

Injections. Diamorphine. Sickness. Sleep.

Something is watching you. Above you it grins and when you wake, it laughs. You wish for something, for someone, to free you from its gaze.

The pain rises and rises and your eyes bulge. When you wake from your dreams, your room is brightly lit. Eerily calm. Lights flicker. You follow the movement of shadows.

Something is here, watching, always. You can feel it.

You press the button. You call out. Nothing. There's no-one. Beyond the door to your room there is only darkness. Outside, the same. Where is everyone? Your breath feels hot.

Breathe in.

The air darkens and hardens. Colours bleed down the walls.

Are you awake?

Suddenly people rush in. A blur of white coats. They dance. Their faces twist and laugh.

Lights flash. Noise. Urgent movements. The hospital corridors spin wildly.

Above you, it is watching. Always.

The morphine pump chirps. It ticks.

Someone grips your hand. Tight. You don't have the strength to squeeze back, but you wish you could.

Around you there is so much noise, but you can't focus. Voices without bodies.

You sleep.

You dream of churches, of your childhood.

A nurse fades into view.

'What's happening?' you ask, feebly.

'You're in intensive care,' she replies. 'You'll be okay. You're doing well.'

She drifts away.

Your arms are crossed against your chest to make the shape of an X. The priest is a waxwork cloaked in white. He waves his arm. You sit down, cold against the ground.

Someone wipes tears from your cheeks but you don't remember crying. These nurses see people cry every day. They see people die every week.

Somewhere in the hospital there are newborn babies, bald and useless. They wail and they cry. They scream. Some of them die.

You awake feeling strange. Like you're under water. You've felt weak before, but not like this. Breathe in. It hurts. Your eyes twitch and your head slumps. A nurse stands watching you, silent. She eyes you carefully, takes your obs. A voice echoes, tells you to get some rest.

Dice tumble. This is a game of odds.

Wait for the plane to crash. Hear the screams and shouts. You're alone.

This scene is yours and only yours. There is no sound above

you, no sound around you, no sound below.
Eyes watch you, unblinking, empty.

Breathe in.
This scene is solitary, but around you it is busy.
Breathe in.
White coats.
Tiredness overcomes you. People around you are smiling. Why? You smile. Outside you can hear the horns and bass of carnival music.
Breathe in.
You sleep.

Wake up. Television and distilled water. You cough and your lungs jangle and gurgle and the pain rises up into your neck and there's blood on the sheets. You look around in the darkness for someone, but no-one's here.

You have no mood. Music is just sound. You feed the cord of your headphones backwards and forwards between your thumb and forefinger like rosary beads, but without prayer.
There's a multi-faith chapel in the hospital, downstairs. When you've been well and walking, you've hobbled past the chapel plenty of times but never gone in. The same few patients go in and out, the same dire expressions on their faces. They too are alone. You walk past each other like ghosts.
The clouds in the early evening sky form shapes like faces. Ominous. Sweat forms on your neck and around your eyes.

You awake and you're dizzy. Your head no longer feels heavy; it feels light – lighter than you've ever felt before. Rising.
Memories of childhood merry-go-rounds whirl past.

Your stomach turns. You feel a quiet panic rise inside you and you cough violently.

'What's happening?' you ask, to no-one.

Those same eyes watch you from above.

The room spirals.

Suddenly there's the shrieking of machines and the red flash of lights in the darkness and the swift movement of animated bodies all around you. Dancing. Dancing.

You hope this is a dream.

You pray.

Blood pounds deafeningly, painfully, in your ears.

Like the marching of feet.

Feet on gravel. A slow mournful crunch. Everyone you know is here. Waiting.

There are so many people in your room.

Frantic shouting.

The lights are bright.

There are noises you don't understand.

Music calls out to you. Your favourite songs. Sombre notes and tones.

You feel so weak. So empty. So tired.

It's almost pleasant.

The oxygen mask tastes like stale breath.

A nurse leans over you with her hand on your arm.

You drift.

The car snakes sluggishly over the gravel with grim solemnity, and through the glass reads your name in flowers of green and white.

She shakes you and you look right up into her eyes.
They're wide.
　She says your name.
　Again and again she says it.
　'You're doing so well,' she says.
　'Just breathe.'
　'Just breathe.'

You breathe in.
　Breathe in.
　Breathe in.
　Breathe.
　Breathe.

He'd have liked it here.

Your parents are older. Elderly. Your mum holds your dad's arm as they stand close together.

Behind them is your sister. You barely recognise her – she's so much older too; she seems tired, but content. Nobody speaks.

Upon silent consensus, the three walk away. They meander through the grass and the flowers turned brittle by frost.

Next they're in a pub you don't recognise. Drunken men cackle and howl in the far distance.

A group of your friends arrive. They've aged too. Some have partners attached to their arms whom you don't recognise.

Drinks are ordered.

Chit-chat.

Crisps.

You hear your name mentioned a couple of times, but most of the talk is of work and family.

The conversation moves on.

Time has not forgotten you but your place within it has faded.

You've become an abstraction. A ghost.

A few people weakly attempt nostalgia, but memory is imperfect, and shared meaning has thinned.

This scene is mild and good-natured.

Soon enough, people start to throw scarves over shoulders and shove fingers into gloves.

There are handshakes and hugs.

And when it's just the three of them left – amongst the litter of the crisp packets and the pint glasses – your mum, dad and sister pause for a moment before getting up to leave.

'He'd have liked it here,' your dad says, to what's left of his family, and to himself.

You watch and you long to reach out and to hold them and laugh and joke with them.

But you know that you can't.

By now you're no more than a stranger.

The fire crackles.

Your dad wraps his arm around your mum and your sister and they amble out the door.

The first number in your phonebook is 'Home'.

This scene is quiet. The low buzz of electricity makes the air sound like faint static. There are no other sounds on the ward.

Your arms are thin and weak. They're spotted with purple blotches. Your skin curls into clumps where it's peeled.

Morphine makes your brain feel water-logged.

Your breath rattles in your chest.

Breathe normally.

You splutter.

Blood and mucus have formed painful crusts and sores around your mouth and nostrils.

It's two weeks since you finished your final dose of chemotherapy. It's several days since you left intensive care. You've been stable since; the last few days were quietly uneventful. You know that soon they might let you go home.

You feel a profound, crippling sense of uncertainty and emptiness.

You hold your phone in your hand, not quite sure why.

The first number in your phonebook is 'Home'.

You go back to sleep.

It's the early hours of the morning and a registrar, instead of a nurse, comes to take your observations. You recognise him as one of the doctors who stayed with you during one of the nights when things got bad. He looks at you thoughtfully as he makes his notes.

You have an urge to ask him, 'What's going to happen?' but you can't bring yourself to say anything at all.

Eventually, he smiles, tells you you're doing well, and leaves.

In the afternoon your support worker comes to visit. She sits by you and speaks softly, gently; she listens patiently, intently, earnestly, as you struggle to answer her questions.

Your breathing feels slow and raw.

She hands you something.

'What does cancer mean to you?' it reads. It's a leaflet for a young persons' cancer support group.

She smiles. 'For when you're feeling a little better. Maybe even after you've gone home. It might be good to meet other young people.'

What does cancer mean to you?

You ask yourself this question after she's gone. Cancer means no one thing to you; it means a thousand moments and memories.

It means baldness. It means nausea and vomit. It means gut infections. Cancer means urine bottles and tissues crusty with dried blood. It means infusions of chemotherapy into your blood and injections of chemotherapy into your spine. Cancer means joylessness where before there was joy: books, TV, films, food, drink, sleep – what they were to you before they are no longer. Cancer means a Hickman line hanging grimly from your chest that makes you feel less like a human and more like a machine. It means a fresh blanket of dead skin in your bedsheets each morning. It means stripping the last dying hairs from your head with a razor as you stare into the reflection of your eyes in the mirror. It means the look of sadness and shock on your grandmother's face and the subsequent warmth of her embrace. Cancer means masturbating into a plastic pot in a fertility clinic so a doctor can freeze your sperm for some day in the future when you might have kids, if you live. Cancer means the taut, strained expressions on the faces of your family, eyes glassy, as they digest the news and internally promise themselves that they'll be strong. It means long nights with only your own frightening mind and the drip-drip-drip of the chemo. It means losing yourself in morphine dreams and swallowing silent screams when you awake to the face of some indescribable evil. Cancer means the waiting game. It means tension. It means numbers and charts. Odds and percentages. Luck and chance. Cancer means saying goodbye to who you were and accepting the truth of who you are: a helpless, desperate, pitiful shadow. It means suspending hope in favour of denial – not fighting, but resisting. Cancer means everything to you now: it is your life.

This time when your parents visit your sister comes too. The air is dense with silence and tension. This scene is all long smiles and longer pauses.

'So good to see you're off the oxygen mask,' your mum offers. 'You must be much more comfortable now.'

You smile. You are. The clip on your nose is subtler, less invasive.

'We're thinking of booking a holiday,' your dad says. 'Somewhere by the sea, with good pubs and nice clean country air.'

His easy smile betrays something you've not seen in his face for a while: a sincere sense of hope.

He believes you'll be okay. Nobody wants to say it, but everyone knows that's what he's thinking.

'That sounds great, Dad.' You can feel yourself welling up so you pretend to be leafing through your pile of old magazines and newspapers.

Your sister is sat closest to you. She rubs your shoulder and smiles. You smile back.

In the days that follow your time in intensive care, a deeply uncomfortable restlessness begins to take hold of you.

You lie in bed and you itch. You turn over and over but you cannot find comfort. Nights blend into days. All feels grey. You fixate on that moment when they will let you go home. You imagine the relief. The release.

If you had the energy you would pace the room; instead you do so in your mind.

As the hours pass by the wait gets harder and you begin to feel like somehow you're crumbling. Your ears fill with a vibrant hum that you can't shake. You relive the worst moments of the last four months again and again in your mind. At night they mingle and merge with your most twisted dreams.

You begin to detach yourself. You think of yourself from the outside. You are no longer the subject, but the object. You watch yourself with dispassionate interest.

What will you do now?

Your consultant visits. He is coy about what is likely to happen when you leave hospital.

'We've had a lot of success with the trial,' he says, obliquely.

'Will I need any more treatment?' you ask.

'That depends. We'll have to do some follow-up treatment as an out-patient… Until the PET scan and bone marrow biopsy, we can't be sure what will happen next.'

Doubt floods your mind. If the treatment hasn't worked, if this has all been for nothing, you don't know that you have the strength to do it all again.

You just want to go home.

'When do you think…?' you try to ask the question but stutter pathetically.

Your consultant takes this in his stride.

'We'll do all we can. Hopefully it won't be any more than a few days now.'

As the hours pass, only one thought occupies your mind: *What if the treatment hasn't worked?*

You think about this as rationally as you can. The treatment you have received is the most aggressive regime of chemotherapy that's available. If the disease hasn't responded, it is unlikely to respond to any similar treatment.

Nothing is certain; this is all a game of odds.

You do feel certain, however, that you cannot do this again. You are spent. Empty. There is no fight left in your body and no courage or pride left in your soul.

You try to be completely honest with yourself and you realise something profoundly empowering: you would rather die than do this again.

This knowledge sits with you like a weapon.

You would rather die than do this again.

The blood and the vomit and the needles and the machines and the darkness and the flashing lights scatter before your eyes and you know that you have given this absolutely everything that you have to give.

All that you want now is to rest. To be with the people you love. To feel the softness of the pillows on the bed you slept in as a child. To hug your mum in the morning. To feel warmth, and love, and dignity.

When the consultant eventually tells you that today is the day you can go home, he catches you by surprise. His tone is casual. Matter-of-fact. Clinical.

The anti-climax pulses around you and you walk backwards and forwards, stepping into nothing and then back again, lost for purpose and motion.

You pick up your phone.

The first number in your phonebook is 'Home'.

You dial and a familiar voice answers and your eyes begin to water.

Afterword

There is no easy ending. No single moment of understanding. No sublime self-awareness. Nothing that makes things any easier.

Cancer is an ugly truth. The bleeding and the shitting and the vomiting and the skin-shedding and the pissing into cardboard bottles. The pain. The shivering. The hopeless, hollow dependency on painkillers. The depression and the counselling. It's unfashionable and uncomfortable.

The physical pain a cancer patient goes through can, for some people, be terrible; the psychological trauma that must be endured can be just as damaging. Each person's experience of cancer and its countless torturous treatments is absolutely individual because everyone's physiology is different and everyone's disease is different. So you're alone – and you know you are. The battle is between you and the evil in your body. There is no isolation like it in the world.

Even now, in the comfort of remission, I carry my cancer with me like a secret. It is mine and mine alone.

I never wanted to be defined by cancer, but thinking that way was naïve. It will always be a vital part of my identity – this is unavoidable – and I wouldn't have it any other way.

It was during those long, dark hospital nights that the seeds of my dreams were sown. I never want to forget who I was in those moments.

I never want to forget the frailty, the pain, the sadness.

Everywhere I go, the boy in the mirror goes with me. He is both a reminder of what I have been through, and a threat of what I may become again.

I see him in shop windows and in the light reflecting from pint glasses and in the eyes of the people I love. He will be with me forever.

I wrote this book to help me heal.

I hope that people will read it, and in some way it will help them too.

And I guess the last paragraph of the last chapter of my book is this: I'm sat at my computer and I finish the crucial last words, on which so much seems to rest, and I step back and I look at the screen and I know I'm supposed to infer some deeper meaning or profound sense of self, but all that happens is I remember the pain and the terror, and the fear that I witnessed written on the faces of the people I love, and the way I saw in my own reflection the slow but tangible erosion of everything that I was; and here and now I can do nothing but exhale deeply and walk lazily to the bathroom, where I stand in front of the mirror and I stare right into the depths of my own eyes, and I see myself not as healthy and older and secure like I am, but young and frail and bald and dying and crying out for help from someone, from anyone, and I see this ghost and all I can do is tell him how sorry I am, and how grateful, and I walk back to my room and fold myself into bed and I dream of hospital corridors and whirring machines and serene windows dotted with silent rain.